English for Medicine

医療・看護のためのやさしい総合英語

Toshiaki Nishihara
Mayumi Nishihara
Assunta Martin

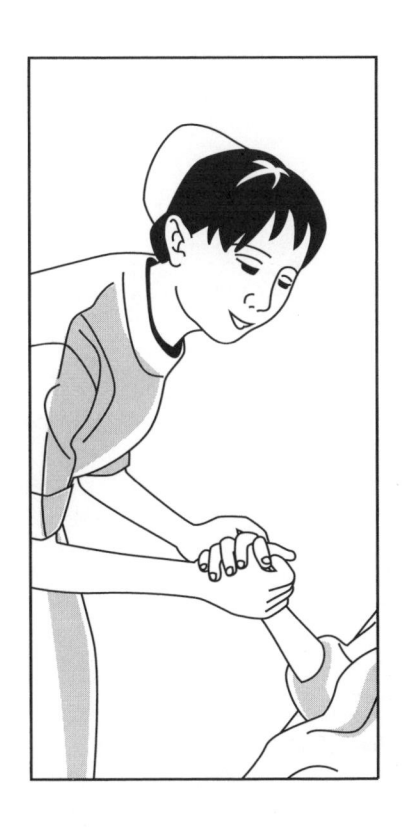

KINSEIDO

Kinseido Publishing Co., Ltd.
3-21 Kanda Jimbo-cho, Chiyoda-ku,
Tokyo 101-0051, Japan

Copyright © 2005 by Toshiaki Nishihara
　　　　　　　　　Mayumi Nishirara
　　　　　　　　　Assunta Martin

All rights reserved. No part of this publication may be reproduced, stored in a retrieval system, or transmitted, in any form or by any means, electronic, mechanical, photocopying, recording or otherwise, without the prior permission of the publisher.

First published 2005 by Kinseido Publishing Co., Ltd.

　　　　　　　　　　　　表紙デザイン：スタジオベゼル
　　　　　　　　　　　　編集協力：めだかスタジオ

は し が き

　本書は、医学部、看護系大学、看護系専門学校などの学生を対象とした英語の授業用テキストです。実際に医療の現場において必要と思われる英会話を想定し、それを学ぶことで英語による基礎的コミュニケーション能力を養うことを目的としています。

　また、専門課程で学ぶこととなる医療英語への橋渡しとなるように工夫されているのも本書の特徴の1つです。各章において専門課程で必要と思われる語彙や情報等をわかりやすくふんだんに紹介しています。

　Reading Exerciseでは、最近話題になっているものを取り上げるとともに、実際に使用されている英文の処方箋や薬品の説明書なども取り入れ、理解を深められるように配慮してあります。各章の最初にあるVocabulary Studyは、Listening ActivityやReading Activityの負担を軽減させるとともに、Brainstormingの役割も担っています。さらに、章の終りにはNotesを付し、英語圏と日本での医療の違い、語法説明等についてふれました。

　テキストの中ほどと最後には、復習テスト（Review Test）を用意し、学習内容の定着を確認できます。巻末には、有益と思われる表現集や人体図も付してあります。付属のCDには、各章で紹介されている英会話をNatural Speed、Slow Speedの順序で収録してありますので、予習・復習に大いにご活用ください。

　このテキストでの学習が、将来、医療関係に従事する学生の一助となれば幸いです。

　なお、本書の内容については、著者の気付かない不備もあると思われます。多くの先生方からのご教示、ご批判をいただければ幸いです。

　最後に、本書の出版に際して、大変お世話になった金星堂の福岡氏と佐藤氏に、心から感謝申し上げます。

著　者

CONTENTS

Chapter 1 ・・・・・・・・・ *7*
Chapter 2 ・・・・・・・・ *11*
Chapter 3 ・・・・・・・・ *15*
Chapter 4 ・・・・・・・・ *19*
Chapter 5 ・・・・・・・・ *23*
Chapter 6 ・・・・・・・・ *27*
Chapter 7 ・・・・・・・・ *31*
● *Review Test 1* ・・・・・・ *35*

Chapter 8 ・・・・・・・・ *39*
Chapter 9 ・・・・・・・・ *43*
Chapter 10 ・・・・・・・ *47*
Chapter 11 ・・・・・・・ *51*
Chapter 12 ・・・・・・・ *55*
Chapter 13 ・・・・・・・ *59*
● *Review Test 2* ・・・・・・ *63*

症状集 /68
表現集 /71
人体図 /74

Chapter 1

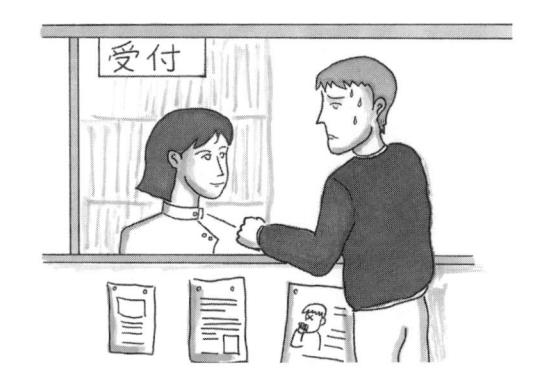

I Vocabulary Study

次にあげる英語表現の意味を表す日本語を選択肢から選んで、その記号を答えなさい。

1. fever   (   )   a. 内科医
2. paralysis   (   )   b. 吐く
3. internist   (   )   c. 熱
4. vomit   (   )   d. 温度・体温
5. temperature   (   )   e. 麻痺

CD 2/3

II Listening Activity

会話文を聞いて、空欄に英語を書き入れなさい。ただし、最初の1回は、テキストの文を見ないで、聞いてください。

Receptionist: Good morning. Do you have an ¹_____ a doctor?

Patient: Sorry, no, I don't.

Receptionist: Are you a ²_____ here?

Patient: No, I'm just visiting the area.

Receptionist: Is this ³_____ to our hospital? May I see ⁴_____?

Patient: Okay.

Receptionist: How are you today?

Patient: I ⁵_____ twice this morning, and I have a ⁶_____. I'd like to have an ⁷_____

	▓▓▓▓▓▓▓▓▓▓▓▓▓▓▓▓▓.
Receptionist:	All right. Could you ⁸▓▓▓▓▓▓▓▓▓▓▓▓▓▓ this form before you see a doctor?
Patient:	Here you are.
Receptionist:	Thank you. Now I'd like to ⁹▓▓▓▓▓▓▓▓▓▓▓ and pulse. What is ¹⁰▓▓▓▓▓▓▓▓▓▓▓▓▓▓▓?
Patient:	96 °F.
Receptionist:	Please wait for a moment until your name is called.

III Reading Activity

次の英文を読んで、設問に答えなさい。

Polio

Polio is a disease caused by a virus. It enters the human body through the mouth. It can cause paralysis and kill people by paralyzing the muscles that help them breathe.

The disease used to be very common in the United States. It killed thousands of people a year before a vaccine was developed for it. In 1916, a polio epidemic in the country killed 6,000 people and paralyzed 27,000 more. In the early 1950s, there were more than 20,000 cases of polio each year. Vaccinations for polio began in 1955. By 1960, the number of cases dropped to about 3,000, and by 1979 there were only about 10 recorded cases.

The polio vaccine is administered in one of two ways: by oral intake of a live, weakened polio vaccine (OPV) or by injection (IPV). Although OPV is still used in many parts of the world, IPV is recommended in the United States today. The recommendation for IPV is based on a medical study that suggests that OPV may actually cause polio. According to this study, one person in 2.4 million risks contracting polio from the OPV vaccine.

■NOTES■
OPV 　毒性を弱めた活性のポリオワクチンを経口摂取すること
IPV 　不活性のポリオワクチンを注射で摂取すること

■Comprehension Questions■

1. How do we get polio?

2. What does polio cause?

3. How can we get immunity to polio?

4. What is an epidemic?

5. What type of polio vaccine is recommended in the United States? Why?

IV Writing Activity
今まで学習した表現を参考にして、次の日本語を英語になおしなさい。

1. 今朝2回ほど吐いて、少々熱があります。

2. 熱と脈を測りたいのですが。

3. 平熱は何度ですか。

V For Your Information

次にあげる病名を調べなさい。

1. Polio
2. Measles
3. Mumps
4. Chickenpox
5. HIV
6. Whooping cough
7. Rubella
8. Diphtheria
9. Hepatitis
10. Tetanus

NOTES

1) 病院などの予約には、make an appointment with を用い、ホテルなどの予約には、reserve/book a single room などのように用います。自分で赴いて、席を確保する場合は、secure the table という表現を用います。

2) アメリカでは、Measles、Mumps、Rubella の頭文字をとって、通称、MMR と呼ばれるワクチンがあります。日本では、これらのワクチンを1種類摂取するとある一定期間をおいて次のワクチンを摂取しますが、アメリカでは3種類を同時に摂取できます。また、MMR と他のワクチンを同時に摂取することも可能です。

3) 日本では摂氏（Celsius）を用いますが、アメリカでは、通例、華氏（Fahrenheit）を用います。これは、ドイツの物理学者の名前に由来し、換算式は、$C = (F - 32) \times 5/9$。

4) 日本では熱を測る際に体温計を脇の下に入れますが、欧米では口の中に体温計を入れることがよくあります。

5) 病院で "How are you?" と尋ねられ、とっさに "Fine." と答える人がいます。これでは、"You don't need to be here." と言われてしまいますから、注意しましょう。

Chapter 2

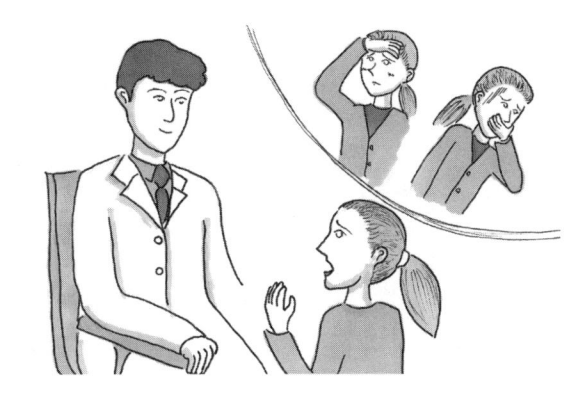

I Vocabulary Study

次にあげる英語表現の意味を表す日本語を選択肢から選んで、その記号を答えなさい。

1. infection   (   )   a. 痛い
2. prescription   (   )   b. 抗生物質
3. antibiotic(s)   (   )   c. （飲み薬の）服用量
4. dose   (   )   d. 処方箋
5. sore   (   )   e. 消毒用の
6. throw up   (   )   f. 吐く
7. antiseptic   (   )   g. 感染

II Listening Activity

会話文を聞いて、空欄に英語を書き入れなさい。ただし、最初の1回は、テキストの文を見ないで、聞いてください。

Nurse: Good morning. I'll take you to the [1]_____.

Patient: Thank you.

Nurse: [2]_____, please.

(*In an examination room*)

Doctor: Good morning. What seems [3]_____?

Patient: I threw up twice this morning, and I have a slight fever. I also have a [4]_____.

Doctor: Can you describe the pain?

Patient: It's a sharp pain.

Doctor: Since when have you had a [5]_____?

Patient: Since last night.
Doctor: What is your normal temperature?
Patient: 97 °F.
Doctor: Now I'd like [6]_____. First, I need to [7]_____ and blood pressure. All right. [8]_____ your sleeve, please. Your heartbeat is quite normal. Take a [9]_____. [10]_____. [11]_____. Now [12]_____ and say "Ah." [13]_____. I recommend these antiseptic lozenges, and they will [14]_____. You need to take antibiotics, too.

III Reading Activity
次の英文を読んで、設問に答えなさい。

Personal Prescription

Patient: Lisa Yamaguchi
Medication: AMOXICILLIN (250 MG/5ML SUSP 150ML)
Directions: Take one teaspoonful by mouth, three times daily for ten days until all is taken.

Common uses:
This medicine is a penicillin-like antibiotic used to treat infections.
How to use this medicine:

Follow the directions for using this medicine provided by your doctor. Shake well before taking a dose. Use a measuring device marked for medicine dosing. Ask your pharmacist for help if you are unsure of how to measure this dose. You may mix this medicine with milk or formula before taking it. If you mix this medicine with milk or formula, use it immediately after mixing. This medicine may be taken on an empty stomach or with food.

Store this medicine at room temperature or in the refrigerator. To clear up your infection completely, continue taking this medicine for the full course of treatment even if you feel better in a few days. Do not miss any doses. If you miss a dose of this medicine, take it as soon as possible. If it is almost time for your next dose, skip the missed dose and go back to your regular dosing schedule. Do NOT take 2 doses at once.

■NOTES■
AMOXICILLIN　アモキシシリン
formula　調合乳

■Comprehension Questions■

1. How many times a day and for how long does a patient need to take the medicine?

2. What is the medicine for?

3. What does s/he need to do before s/he takes the medicine?

4. When you mix the medicine with milk, what do you need to do?

5. When does s/he need to skip a dose of this medicine?

IV Writing Activity
今まで学習した表現を参考にして、次の日本語を英語になおしなさい。

1. 今日はどのような具合ですか。

2. いつから微熱が続いていますか。

3. 深呼吸をしてください。吸って。はいて。

V For Your Information
次にあげる病名または、語句を調べなさい。

1. abdominal pain
2. anemia
3. cerumen
4. abrasion
5. asthma
6. nausea/nauseous
7. acne
8. bronchitis
9. colic
10. allergic reaction
11. burn
12. concussion

NOTES

1) 日本で処方される薬の多くは、「食後」の指定が多く見られますが、アメリカ・イギリスでは、指定された回数を守れば、必ずしも食後にとる必要はありません。ただし、胃腸に不快な感じがある場合には、食後に服用することが薦められています。処方された薬はきちんと最後まで服用し続けることが明記されています。

2) 食前に必ず処方する薬の1つに、**FOSAMAX**と呼ばれるものがあります。これは更年期の女性用で、カルシウムやミネラルを含むものです。

Chapter 3

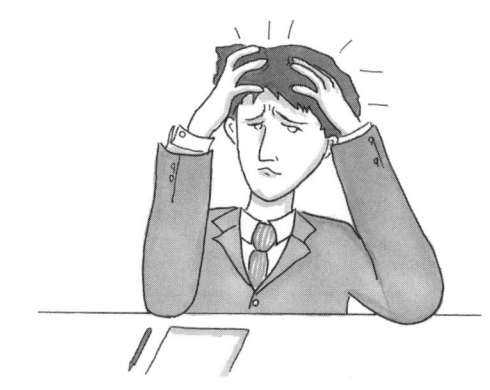

I　Vocabulary Study

次にあげる英語表現の意味を表す日本語を選択肢から選んで、その記号を答えなさい。

1. itchy　　　　　　　　（　）　a. 偏頭痛
2. migraine headache　　（　）　b. 鼻がつまった
3. stuffy nose　　　　　　（　）　c. 軽くする・和らげる
4. throbbing　　　　　　（　）　d. ずきずきする
5. relieve　　　　　　　　（　）　e. かゆい

CD 6/7

II　Listening Activity

会話文を聞いて、空欄に英語を書き入れなさい。ただし、最初の1回は、テキストの文を見ないで、聞いてください。

Doctor:　　[1]_____ here today?

Patient:　　I have a migraine headache.

Doctor:　　Is it localized [2]_____ of your head? Does it [3]_____ in bright light?

Patient:　　The headache is located here.

Doctor:　　[4]_____?

Patient:　　It is dull and throbbing.

Doctor:　　Is it bad enough [5]_____?

Patient:　　Yes, the pain wakes me up at night.

Doctor:　　Is it continuous or does it [6]_____?

Patient:　　It's continuous.

Doctor: Is there anything that ⁷_____?
Patient: The pain is relieved by lying down.

III Reading Activity
次の英文を読んで、設問に答えなさい。

Hay Fever

Hay fever is not associated with a true fever, but describes allergic rhinitis, which is an inflammation of the nasal passages caused by an allergic reaction. Allergic symptoms may appear when we are exposed to:

i)   Pollens (seasonal allergic rhinitis)
ii) Dust, animal dander, or feathers (perennial rhinitis)
iii) Changes in temperature, cold air, air pollutants, and oral contraceptives (vasomotor rhinitis)

Tobacco smoke, and heavily polluted air can worsen the symptoms. Symptoms include frequent sneezing, itchy or watery eyes, runny or stuffy nose, and itching in the roof of the mouth. If hay fever is a problem for you, it is recommended that you have immunotherapy, which involves injection of allergen extracts to change your body's response to the allergens, thereby reducing symptoms.

■NOTES■
seasonal allergic rhinitis　季節特有の花粉がもとで生じるアレルギー的な鼻炎
dander　動物の皮膚や毛からでるふけ
perennial rhinitis　年間を通して、ほこり、ふけ、羽がもとで生じる鼻炎
vasomotor rhinitis　気温の変化、空気中の汚染物質などがもとで生じる鼻炎
immunotherapy　免疫療法

■ Comprehension Questions ■

1. What is "hay fever"?

2. Describe three types of hay fever.

3. Describe the symptoms of hay fever.

4. What worsens the symptoms?

5. If you are suffering from hay fever, what should you try?

IV Writing Activity
今まで学習した表現を参考にして、次の日本語を英語になおしなさい。

1. 偏頭痛がします。

2. 頭の一方に見られる局所的な痛みですか。

3. 持続性のある痛みですか。それとも、ときおり生じる痛みですか。

V For Your Information
次にあげる病名または、語句を調べなさい。

1. constipation
2. eczema
3. dehydration
4. contact dermatitis
5. anthrax
6. diarrhea
7. contusion
8. enuresis
9. dislocation
10. croup
11. epilepsy
12. food allergy

NOTES

1) 花粉症といってもそれを引き起こす原因となる植物が国によって異なります。日本では、すぎ花粉（cedar pollen）が花粉症を引き起こす主な原因の1つですが、アメリカでは、ブタクサの花粉（通称ragweed pollen）が主な原因の1つです。人口の15-20％近くの人が花粉症に苦しむイギリスでは、ライ麦（Rye）、牧草としてのヒロハナウシノケグサ（meadow fescue）などが原因であるようです。また、イギリスでは、湿疹や喘息など、アトピー性のもの（atopic conditions）が見られる家系では、花粉症にかかる可能性が高いことが知られています。

2) 花粉症の症状を抑えるものとして、アメリカでも抗ヒスタミン剤がよく使用されますが、その他には、鼻詰まりを緩和する錠剤（decongestant tablet）やスプレーが処方されます。また、お医者さんからは、ドラッグストアにあるスプレー（over-the-counter nose sprays）を長期にわって使用すると症状を悪化させる可能性が高いことが説明されます。ドラッグストアにある薬のことを over-the-counter drugs と呼びます。

3) 薬によっては、1度に服用できる量や1日に服用できる量などに注意が与えられている場合があるので注意が必要です。

　　（例）　Do not take more than 1 at any one time.
　　　　　　Do not take more than 8 in 24 hours.

Chapter 4

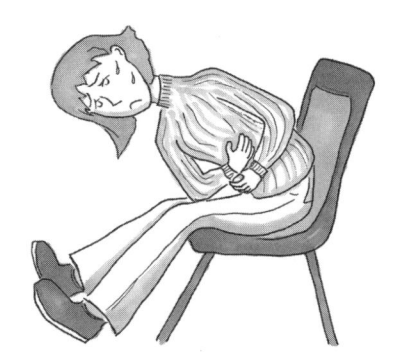

I Vocabulary Study
次にあげる英語表現の意味を表す日本語を選択肢から選んで、その記号を答えなさい。

1. artery / arteries （　）   a. むくみ・腫れること
2. abdomen （　）   b. 肝炎
3. liver disease （　）   c. 大便
4. bloating （　）   d. 腹部
5. stool （　）   e. 動脈

CD 8/9

II Listening Activity
会話文を聞いて、空欄に英語を書き入れなさい。ただし、最初の1回は、テキストの文を見ないで、聞いてください。

Doctor: Good morning. [1]_____ you here today?

Patient: I have some pains, sharp pains around here. (*Pointing to her abdomen and groin*)

Doctor: All right. I'd like to examine you now. Would you like to [2]_____ on your back? I'll take a look at your stomach. [3]_____. [4]_____.

Patient: I'm in pain.

Doctor: Does anything worsen your pain?

Patient: I'm in pain. I'm in pain.

Doctor: [5]_____. I'm going to [6]_____, too. That's it. We're finished. I think there's [7]_____ with one of your arteries because of your high blood pressure.

III Reading Activity

次の英文を読んで、設問に答えなさい。

(Anti-Diarrheal/Anti-gas)

Uses: controls the symptoms of diarrhea plus bloating, pressure, and cramps commonly referred to as gas.

Directions: See the chart below for the correct dose:
Chew the first dose and take with water after the first loose stool.
If needed, chew the next dose and take with water after the next loose stool.
Drink plenty of clear liquids to prevent dehydration.

Dosage	Age	First dose	Next dose	Maximum number per day
Adults	12yrs and over	2 tablets ●●	1 tablet ●	4 tablets ●●●●
Children	9-11yrs (60-95 lbs)	1 tablet ●	1/2 tablet ◗	3 tablets ●●●
Children	6-8yrs (48-59 lbs)	1 tablet ●	1/2 tablet ◗	2 tablets ●●

WARNINGS

Do Not Use if:
- You have a high fever (over 101 °F)
- Blood or mucus is in your stool
- You have had a rash or other allergic reaction.

Do Not Use Without Asking A Doctor
- For more than 2 days
- If you are taking antibiotics
- If you have a history of liver disease

As with any drug, if you are pregnant or nursing a baby, seek the advice of a health professional before using this product.

■NOTES■
lb / lbs（複数）　　重量の単位を表すラテン語のlibra(e)に由来する。pound(s)を表す記号

■Comprehension Questions■

1. What is the medicine for?

2. Can a four-year old child take the medicine?

3. What should we do to prevent dehydration?

4. When can't you take the medicine?

5. Can a pregnant woman take the medicine without asking a doctor?

IV Writing Activity
今まで学習した表現を参考にして、次の日本語を英語になおしなさい。

1. 仰向けに寝ていただけますか。

2. 脱水症状がおきないように、沢山の水分をとって下さい。

3. 血便や粘液がみられる場合には、この薬は用いないでください。

V For Your Information

次にあげる病名を調べなさい。

1. gastroenteritis
2. insomnia
3. scabies
4. headache
5. laryngitis
6. scarlet fever
7. herpangina
8. dyspepsia
9. sinusitis
10. impetigo
11. hypertension
12. tonsillitis

NOTES

1) 日本では、休日診療がどこで行われているのかを消防署に連絡して知ることができます。しかしながら、アメリカで911に電話すると、緊急事態ととられ、叱られることになります。緊急な場合は、近くに総合病院がある場合は、Emergencyというところに行くようにしましょう。

2) 脱水症状など緊急を要する場合を除いては、下痢症状でEmergencyへ行っても、看護師による問診と触診で終わる場合があります。問診と触診だけでもEmergencyを利用すると数百ドルの請求をされますので、症状を十分に見てかかるようにしましょう。乳児の場合、下痢の場合に飲ませるミルクと薬がドラッグストアで入手できます。

3) 幼児語で大便のことは、poo-poo、小便のことは、pee-peeと表現されます。医学用語では、それぞれstool、urineと表現されます。

（例） I need a stool/urine sample.

Chapter 5

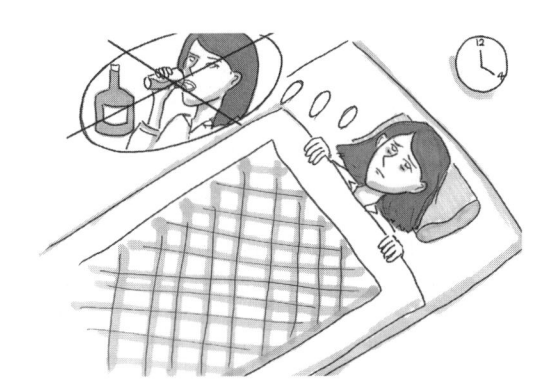

I Vocabulary Study
次にあげる英語表現の意味を表す日本語を選択肢から選んで、その記号を答えなさい。

1. anxious   (　) a. 気持ちを落ちつかせる
2. depression   (　) b. うつ・憂鬱
3. frantic   (　) c. 鎮静剤
4. handle   (　) d. 広がり
5. calm down   (　) e. 不安・心配して
6. prevalence   (　) f. 対処する
7. sedative   (　) g. ひどく興奮した・気が狂いそうな

II Listening Activity
会話文を聞いて、空欄に英語を書き入れなさい。ただし、最初の1回は、テキストの文を見ないで、聞いてください。

Doctor:　Good to see you again. How can I help you?

Patient:　I've been having [1]_____ for the past three or four weeks. I feel exhausted in the morning.

Doctor:　Is [2]_____ you?

Patient:　Yes. Our son, Derek, has been having some trouble in school.

Doctor:　I understand. Is [3]_____ you?

Patient:　Well. . . , I'm also a little frantic about a deadline for an important project that I need to complete by December. I've been working [4]_____ and late every night.

Doctor: How are you handling this stress?
Patient: I usually have two or three drinks to calm down.
Doctor: Oh, that's not a good idea. Alcohol is one of the most common ⁵_____. It would be much better if you had a warm bath and read a novel before going to sleep. In your case, I don't think you are suffering from depression or a medical condition. Come see me ⁶_____ if your sleep doesn't improve. I don't think you need a prescription for a sedative.

III Reading Activity
次の英文を読んで、設問に答えなさい。

Sleeping Problems

According to a new Gallup poll released recently, nearly half of U.S adults, or 87 million people suffer from sleep-related problems. They have difficulty sleeping. Some are suffering from insomnia, which is defined as any severe problem falling asleep or staying asleep. Many Americans are tense, anxious or worried about things like work or their family. In addition to stress in the workplace and families, the frantic pace of modern society is leaving more Americans awake. New statistics show that 43% of people have occasional or frequent insomnia cited as the primary cause. The prevalence of occasional insomnia increased from 27 % in 1991 to 35 % in 1995. Many people do not think that sleeplessness is a big enough problem to be concerned about. What is worse, since many people do not think sleeplessness is a serious problem, they are reluctant to seek professional help.

■NOTES■
Gallup poll　ギャロップの世論調査

■Comprehension Questions■

1. How many people suffer from sleep-related problems in the U.S?

2. What exactly is the problem?

3. What is the definition of insomnia?

4. What are some of the causes of insomnia?

5. According to the passage, what makes the situation worse?

IV Writing Activity
今まで学習した表現を参考にして、次の日本語を英語になおしなさい。

1. 不眠症とは、なかなか寝付けず、睡眠状態が持続しない深刻な状態をいう。

2. 多くの人が睡眠を十分にとれないことで苦しんでいる。

3. 多くの人は、不眠は気にかけるような重要な問題だと考えていない。

V For Your Information

次の英文の意味を日本語になおしなさい。

1. What is the medication used for?
2. How does the medication work?
3. Should I take the medicine with or without food?
4. What are the side effects of this medication?
5. How long will it be before I notice the effects of this medication?
6. How long do I need to take this medication for?
7. Are there any precautions I should take while on this medication?
8. What do I do if I miss a dose?
9. How should I store this medication?
10. Can I drink alcohol while taking this medication?

NOTES

1) come see you という表現は、口語表現です。come to see you、come and see you とも言います。come see you は、"Did you come see me?" "I should come see you." のように、come に語尾変化が生じていない場合にのみ用いられます。類例として、"Go get it." があります。

2) アメリカでは、hypnosedatives と呼ばれる睡眠誘発剤を飲む人が多くいますが、長期にわたる使用は副作用（side-effects）をともないます。

3) 寝つきが悪い場合、アメリカでは、寝る前に糖分を含んだ食べ物や飲み物を控えるようにアドバイスしています。また、睡眠のパターンには個人差がありますから、他人と比べないようにアドバイスしています。さらに、リラックスするための1つの手段として、読書やゆっくりお風呂につかること（have a soak in the bath）などを勧めています。日本人にとってはお風呂でゆったりした気分を楽しむのはふつうのことですので、習慣の違いが見てとれます。

4) 時差などによって生じる不眠は、circadian rhythm disorder と呼ばれています。心身ともに疲れ、やる気がない状態を nervous breakdown と言います。

5) 最近の調査によると、健康な人が1日1杯のワインを飲むと良いことが報告されています。特に、女性の場合、ワインを1日1杯飲む人は、飲まない人に比べて、心臓病にかかる割合が50％も少ないことが報告されています。しかしながら、妊娠中の人（pregnant women）やこれから妊娠を考えている人（women trying to conceive）は飲酒を控えなくてはいけません。

Chapter 6

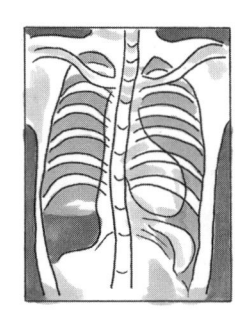

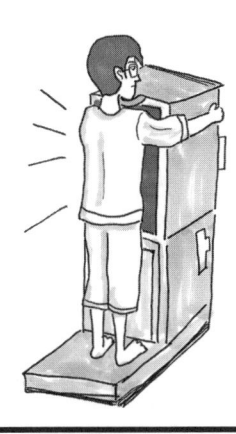

I Vocabulary Study

次にあげる英語表現の意味を表す日本語を選択肢から選んで、その記号を答えなさい。

1. acute   (   )   a. 痰
2. anesthetic   (   )   b. レントゲン写真
3. phlegm   (   )   c. 急性の
4. respiratory   (   )   d. 麻酔剤
5. X-ray   (   )   e. 呼吸器に関する

CD 12/13

II Listening Activity

会話文を聞いて、空欄に英語を書き入れなさい。ただし、最初の1回は、テキストの文を見ないで、聞いてください。

Doctor: We'll have to do [1]_____ to find out what's causing your problem. We need to get your [2]_____. Also, for two days running, I'd like you to [3]_____ of the phlegm and sputum that you cough up in the morning. We will be sending the sample off to the lab for testing. [4]_____ if you have any particular germs present. Following that, you need to have a bronchoscopy done. It's not a [5]_____, but don't worry.

Patient: Does it hurt?

Doctor: You'll be given an anesthetic spray to numb your throat before we begin. It doesn't take more than a few minutes.

Patient: Will I be able to eat anything afterwards?

Doctor: You'll have to wait until the anesthetic has worn off.

■NOTES■

bronchoscopy　気管支鏡法

III Reading Activity

次の英文を読んで、設問に答えなさい。

SARS

SARS (Severe Acute Respiratory Syndrome) was first reported in Asia in February 2003, and the outbreak of SARS continued to spread. The illness spread to more than two dozen countries in North America, South America, Europe, and Asia. More than eight thousand people worldwide became infected with the disease; 813 died.

According to the World Health Organization, SARS is a viral respiratory illness caused by a corona virus. In general, SARS begins with a high fever (temperature greater than 100.4 °F). Other symptoms are headache, a feeling of discomfort, body aches, and diarrhea. After 2 to 7 days, the patient may develop a dry cough and pneumonia.

The virus that causes SARS is thought to be contagious and readily transmitted. If an infected person coughs or sneezes, the droplets from the infected person are propelled a short distance (generally up to 3 feet) through the air and may be deposited on the mucous membranes of the mouth, nose, or eyes of persons who are nearby. The virus can also spread when a person touches a surface or an object contaminated with infectious droplets and then touches his or her mouth, nose, or eye(s). In order to keep from being exposed to the virus, you should follow the instructions below:

> 1) Limit your activities outside the home if SARS cases are reported.
> 2) Wash your hands often and well.
> 3) Cover your mouth and nose with a mask when you go out.

■NOTES■
SARS　重症急性呼吸器症候群
World Health Oraganization（WHO）　世界保健機関

■Comprehension Questions■

1. What is SARS?

2. What are the symptoms of SARS?

3. Is SARS contagious?

4. Describe how the virus spreads.

5. How can we avoid catching this illness?

Ⅳ Writing Activity
今まで学習した表現を参考にして、次の日本語を英語になおしなさい。

1. その検査の前に麻酔スプレーが渡されます。

2. その男の子は発熱した。

3. その病気は、感染した人がくしゃみや咳をすると感染すると考えられている。

V For Your Information

次にあげる病名または、語句を調べなさい。

1. obesity
2. pancreatitis
3. blood transfusion
4. mercy killing
5. contagious disease
6. transplant
7. abortion
8. ulcer
9. heart attack
10. critical condition
11. apoplexy
12. kidney problems

NOTES

1) SARSに続いて、鳥インフルエンザ（avian influenza/bird flu）が問題になっていますが、人から人への感染は、human-to-human transmissionやhuman species contaminationと表現されています。また、感染力が強いという意味で、virulent disease、contagious(ness)という表現が用いられています。診断方法が確立していないところでは、pneumonia（肺炎）、dengue fever（デング熱）と診断され、子供が亡くなるというケースもあるようです。最近話題になっているもう1つの病気に狂牛病BSE（Bovine Spongiform Encephalopathy）があります。通称は、mad cow diseaseです。

2) 口内炎は、ある和英辞書によるとstomatitisと記されていますが、この用語では通じない場合があります。その際には、mouth ulcerと表現してみましょう。口唇炎はcheilitis、舌炎はglossitisと言います。

Chapter 7

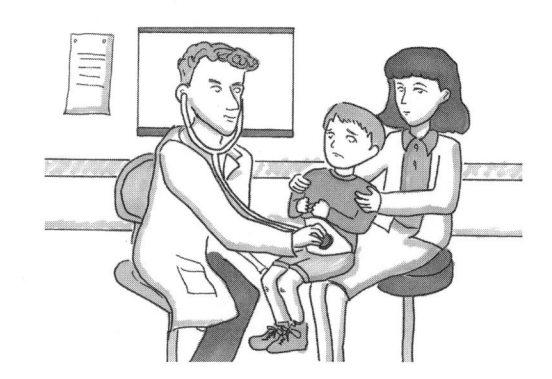

I Vocabulary Study

次にあげる英語表現の意味を表す日本語を選択肢から選んで、その記号を答えなさい。

1. diabetes   (   )   a. 腎臓
2. kidney   (   )   b. 脈管
3. monitor   (   )   c. 糖尿病
4. susceptible   (   )   d. （一定期間）注意深く調べる
5. vessels   (   )   e. 感染しやすい・影響を受けやすい

CD 14/15

II Listening Activity

会話文を聞いて、空欄に英語を書き入れなさい。ただし、最初の１回は、テキストの文を見ないで、聞いてください。

Doctor: Now can I have a look at you [1]_____ where your problem is coming from? Would you like to stay sitting on Mummy's knee? I'm going to put this thing [2]_____. It might be a bit cold.

Boy: I have done this lots of times.

Doctor: Good. Tom, I need a sample of your pee-pee.
(*In the examination room*)

Doctor: The trouble is that you are not making a substance that you need to control the amount of sugar [3]_____. We call this diabetes. If you have too much sugar or too little sugar, it will

	⁴_____ very sick. We need to work on controlling the amount of sugar in your blood. You need to ⁵_____ of insulin.
Boy's mother:	Will that be difficult to do? Can we figure it out?
Doctor:	Not so difficult. The nurse will show you ⁶_____.

III Reading Activity
次の英文を読んで、設問に答えなさい。

Diabetes

A recent health study done in Leeds, Britain has observed a noticeable increase of obesity in primary school children. One in five nine-year olds and one in three eleven-year old girls are overweight. Some over-weight school children have diabetes.

Diabetes is a serious problem in young children nowadays. If you have diabetes, your kidneys will be especially susceptible to damage (diabetic nephropathy). Regular monitoring of your kidneys for signs of damage is necessary to take steps to prevent or delay complications. One way to check for damage is a urine microalbumin test. A urine microalbumin test measures the amount of albumin (al-BU-min) in your urine. Albumin is a type of protein that is normally present in high amounts in the bloodstream. The presence of albumin is often the first sign of early kidney damage.

When you have diabetes, it's easy to become focused on the ups and downs of your blood sugar. However, it's also important to pay particular attention to what's happening to your blood vessels. That's mainly because diabetes poses a major threat to your cardiovascular system, putting you at increased risk of having a heart attack or stroke.

■NOTES■
  Leeds　リーズ。イギリス中西部の都市
  nephropathy　腎障害
  albumin　アルブミン。細胞・体液中の単純たん白質

■Comprehension Questions■

1. What is a serious health problem of school children these days?

2. What is susceptible to damage when you have diabetes?

3. What is albumin?

4. What is an early sign of diabetes?

5. In addition to kidney damage, what else does diabetes pose a threat to?

IV Writing Activity
今まで学習した表現を参考にして、次の日本語を英語になおしなさい。

1. お母さんのお膝にすわってくれますか。

2. 問題がどこから来ているか調べるために、診察させてね。

3. 血中の糖分の量をコントロールしないといけないね。

V For Your Information

次にあげる病名または、語句を調べなさい。

1. coronary arteries
2. genitourinary system
3. bowel movement
4. nutrition
5. chronic disease
6. alimentary system
7. appetite
8. tumors
9. cystitis
10. atopic eczema
11. cirrhosis
12. coma

NOTES

1) アメリカでは、30億（3 billion）のピザが消費されています。肥満を防止するなどの健康志向（health conscious）から、炭水化物（carbohydrates）をそれほどとらずに、高たんぱく質（high-protein）を摂取しようとする人たち用のピザが検討されています。炭水化物をそれほどとらない人のことをlow-carb dietersとかcarovoidsと呼びます。

2) 炭水化物（carbohydrates）を多く摂取している女性は、結腸と直腸に見られる癌（colorectal cancer）にかかる危険性が高いことがアメリカで報告されています。colorectalというのは、colon（結腸）とrectum（直腸）の両方に関わるという意味です。結腸・直腸癌の場合、小さなポリープ（Polyps（adeuomas））が5年から15年で癌腫瘍（cancerous tumor）になります。クッキーやケーキ、それにすぐに消化されやすい食べ物（quickly digested foods）を摂取する人では、炭水化物が糖として体内に取り込まれたことを示す値（glycemic index）が高い傾向にあります。玄米（brown rice）などは、体内に取り込むのに時間がかかる炭水化物を含むことから好まれてきているようです。

3) 子供を診察する場合には、英語ではtummyのような幼児語を交えて話をします。

4) 日本では、耳垢がたまると耳鼻咽喉科でとってもらいますが、アメリカでは、小児科（pediatrics）でとってもらいます。また、ドラッグストアで耳垢（ear wax / cerumen）をとるお薬を買い求めることもできます。

Review Test 1

Part 1 LISTENING EXAM

英文を聞き、次の質問に答えなさい。

■■■ Comprehension Questions ■■■

1. Mrs. Lewis ate out for dinner the night before coming to the doctor.
   A. True   B. False
2. Mrs. Lewis has food poisoning.
   A. True   B. False
3. The doctor thinks Mrs. Lewis has the flu.
   A. True   B. False
4. The doctor took Mrs. Lewis' temperature.
   A. True   B. False
5. Mrs. Lewis could pass the flu to other people.
   A. True   B. False
6. The doctor did not give Mrs. Lewis a prescription for medicine.
   A. True   B. False
7. The doctor told Mrs. Lewis to stay home and not go to work.
   A. True   B. False
8. The doctor wants to see Mrs. Lewis again on Tuesday.
   A. True   B. False

Part 2 READING EXAM

次の英文を読んで、設問に答えなさい。

Vitamin D

Vitamin D is a naturally occurring vitamin in a limited number of foods. It is also produced when our skin is exposed to sunlight. It is essential to our health because it allows our bodies to absorb the calcium that we need to keep our bones strong. Recent research indicates that vitamin D may also play an important role in preventing various diseases, diabetes, and hypertension. People with liver and kidney diseases show a marked deficiency in Vitamin D levels. Vitamin D deficiency is caused by poor diet and lack of exposure to sunlight. A deficiency of Vitamin D may result in osteoporosis, which in turn leads to bone loss.

Vitamin D occurs naturally in such foods as salmon and other oily fish, and eggs. Milk, cereals, and yogurts are often fortified with extra Vitamin D. Until recently, physicians believed that adults had less need for Vitamin D than did children, whose bones were not as yet fully formed. This assumption is being questioned now. According to the Harvard Women's Health Watch, a publication by Harvard Medical School, research at Boston's Massachusetts General Hospital discovered that 57% of the people hospitalized were deficient in adequate amounts of Vitamin D. An inexpensive way to get Vitamin D is to sit in sunlight for a few minutes, two or three times a week. Some physicians think that the surest way to get enough Vitamin D is to take a daily supplement.

■NOTES■

Harvard Women's Health Watch ハーバード大学医学部が刊行している情報誌の1つで女性の健康に関わる情報を提供するもの。男性向けの情報誌としてHarvard Men's Health Watch がある
Harvard Medical School ハーバード大学医学部
Boston's Massachusetts General Hospital ボストンにあるマサチューセッツ総合病院

■■■ **Comprehension Questions** ■■■

1. Vitamin D is a vitamin that naturally occurs in _____.
    A. oily fish
    B. broccoli
    C. wheat
    D. oranges
2. Vitamin D is essential for the growth of _____.
    A. hair
    B. nails
    C. healthy bones
    D. beautiful skin
3. We can infer that osteoporosis causes _____.
    A. weight loss
    B. weight gain
    C. kidney disease
    D. bone loss
4. If milk or yogurt is "fortified" with Vitamin D, this means that the milk or yogurt has had Vitamin D _____.
    A. removed   B. added
5. Researchers and doctors now believe that adults do not require or need as much Vitamin D as children.
    A. True   B. False
6. A recent study of hospitalized patients in the US indicated that _____.
    A. less than 50% were deficient in Vitamin D
    B. everyone tested had high amounts of Vitamin D
    C. only slightly more than 40% of the patients were not deficient in Vitamin D
    D. 57% of the patients in the hospital were tested for Vitamin D
7. A few minutes of sun exposure a couple of times a week can increase your levels of Vitamin D.
    A. True   B. False
8. We can infer that a person who seldom goes outside and rarely eats fish, eggs, or fortified cereals may _____.
    A. be deficient in Vitamin D
    B. get enough Vitamin D by eating lots of vegetables
    C. have very strong bones
    D. not need Vitamine D

9. The cheapest way to get enough Vitamin D is to sit in sunlight for thirty minutes every day.
    A. True   B. False
10. Some doctors advise people to take a daily supplement of Vitamin D.
    A. True   B. False

Part 3 VOCABULARY EXAM

1〜10の英文に合う最も適切な語句を選択肢から選んで、答えなさい。

a. insomnia	b. epidemic	c. vaccine
d. prescription	e. acne	f. relieve
g. migraine	h. pulse	i. dose
j. laryngitis	k. nauseous	l. symptoms

1. Can you describe the _____ you have? Do you have a fever, for example?
2. When Susy was a teenager, she ate a lot of fried food and suffered from terrible _____ on her face.
3. Mr. Ueno was very worried about losing his job. Because he slept so poorly, his doctor recommended he take medication for his _____.
4. The teacher was unable to raise her voice or talk with her students because she had _____.
5. The doctor was surprised that the patient's _____ was so rapid.
6. Mrs. Jenkins forgot to take her evening _____ of her antibiotic, so she called her doctor to ask what to do.
7. The pharmacist filled the doctor's _____ and gave the patient instructions on how to take the medicine.
8. The newspapers were filled with articles and information about the SARS _____ that was spreading through China.
9. The ice packs helped to _____ the pain of her sprained ankle.
10. The polio _____ can be administered orally or by injection.
11. Although the young child felt _____, she didn't vomit on the train.
12. I have a _____ headache. It is killing me.

Chapter 8

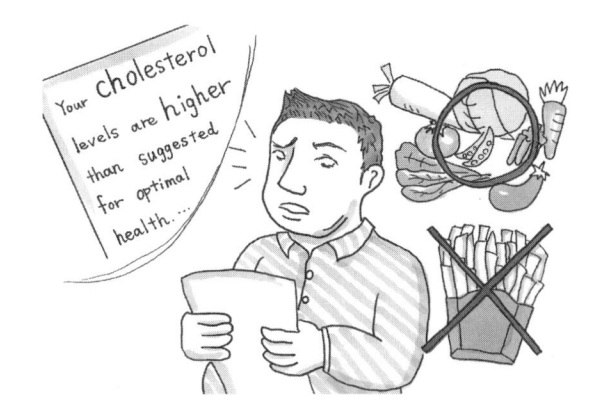

I Vocabulary Study

次にあげる英語表現の意味を表す日本語を選択肢から選んで、その記号を答えなさい。

1. tissue   (   )   a. 検査・健康診断
2. nutrient   (   )   b. 組織
3. checkup   (   )   c. 栄養分（素）
4. cholesterol   (   )   d. 最善な・ベストな
5. lethargic   (   )   e. けだるい・（異常な程）眠い
6. optimal   (   )   f. コレステロール
7. urinalysis   (   )   g. 尿検査・尿分析

CD 17/18

II Listening Activity

会話文を聞いて、空欄に英語を書き入れなさい。ただし、最初の1回は、テキストの文を見ないで、聞いてください。

Doctor:　Good morning. What can I do for you today?

Patient:　I've been feeling tired and lethargic lately. I wonder if it's time for a checkup.

Doctor:　When was [1]_____?

Patient:　About one and a half years ago.

Doctor:　OK. Let me check your [2]_____. Hmmm. It's a little high. Your blood pressure is 130 over 80.

Patient:　Oh, that is higher than normal.

Doctor:　You need to [3]_____ and urine test today.

Patient:　OK.

(Later)

Doctor: Good news. Your urinalysis showed up clear, but your blood test shows that your cholesterol levels are higher than suggested for optimal health. Your [4]_____ is 232.

Patient: Oh no. What should I do?

Doctor: Your LDL levels are high. You need to change your diet and [5]_____. You also need to start a regular exercise routine. [6]_____ vegetables and fruit. [7]_____ deep-fried foods.

Patient: Thanks, Doctor. No more hamburgers and fries for me!

III Reading Activity

次の英文を読んで、設問に答えなさい。

Arterial Diseases

The cardiovascular system is responsible for the marvelous system in our bodies whereby nutrients and proteins are delivered to our tissues and organs, and waste products are removed. Nutrients are carried by our blood through arteries that network throughout the human body. A healthy artery is smooth and elastic, allowing the easy circulation of blood.

The leading causes of death in the United States are heart disease and strokes. If the arteries that supply blood to the heart become clogged with plaque, the passageway through the arteries becomes narrowed. This dangerous condition may result in the formation of a blood clot, which will block the flow of blood in the coronary artery to the heart muscle. The accompanying chest pain is called angina. A stroke may occur when arteries to the brain are blocked, causing a clot to form.

A patient with high cholesterol or high blood pressure is at risk for arterial disease. In order to prevent further damage, a physician will recommend a change in diet and lifestyle in order to reduce cholesterol buildup. In some cases, drugs may be prescribed to help lower blood pressure or cholesterol levels. The surgical procedure known as angioplasty is used in more serious cases to open blocked arteries or to bypass them.

■NOTES■
- plaque　プラーク、血栓
- clot　血のかたまり
- angioplasty　脈間形成、血管形成（術）

■Comprehension Questions■

1. What is the purpose of the cardiovascular system?

2. What causes narrowing of the arteries?

3. What causes blood clots to form?

4. What are the three serious illnesses that may develop as a result of clogged arteries?

5. What advice would a doctor give a patient with arterial disease?

IV Writing Activity
今まで学習した表現を参考にして、次の日本語を英語になおしなさい。

1. 前回健康診断を受けられたのはいつですか。

2. 血液検査と尿検査を受ける必要があります。

3. コレステロール値が、適格とされている値より高いので、脂肪分が多く含まれる食品や牛肉、乳製品の摂取を減らす必要があります。

V For Your Information

次にあげる病名または、語句を調べなさい。

1. acupuncture
2. endorphin
3. melanoma
4. gargle
5. gingivitis
6. benign
7. carcinogen
8. hyperglycemia
9. dilator
10. dialysis

NOTES

1) アメリカ人の多くは、昼食にチーズバーガー、フライドポテト、Lサイズの炭酸飲料（carbonated drink）をとることが多く、そのことが原因で肥満になっているとの指摘があります。肥満により、年間多くの人々が亡くなっています。また、ファーストフードの取りすぎがもとで健康を害し、マクドナルドを訴えたという事例もあります。アメリカのウェストバージニア州では、肥満の人が多く、胃のバイパス手術を受け、健康を取り戻そうとしている人々も多くいます。

2) マクドナルドの超特大サイズのフライドポテトは、29グラムの脂肪分が含まれ、610カロリーにもなります。

3) アルコール分を含まない清涼飲料（soft drink）の自動販売機（vending machine）が各学校に置かれていましたが、最近では、子ども達の健康を守るという理由から撤去されてきています。アメリカでは、自動販売機でアルコール類やタバコの販売は行われていません。

4) 英語でjuiceというと100％果汁のものを指します。オレンジの絞り立てのものをだすお店では、fresh-squeezed juiceという表現がよく見られます。

Chapter 9

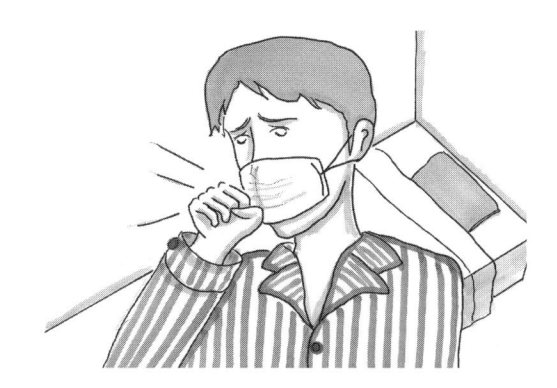

I Vocabulary Study

次にあげる英語表現の意味を表す日本語を選択肢から選んで、その記号を答えなさい。

1. insurance   (　)   a. 治療法
2. thermometer   (　)   b. 体温計・温度計
3. jaundice   (　)   c. 診断
4. remedies   (　)   d. 保険
5. exhaustion   (　)   e. ひどい疲れ
6. diagnosis   (　)   f. 病気がたどる経過に関する医学上の見
7. prognosis   (　)   通し
                          g. 黄疸の

CD 19/20

II Listening Activity

会話文を聞いて、空欄に英語を書き入れなさい。ただし、最初の1回は、テキストの文を見ないで、聞いてください。

Nurse:　　Good morning, Mr. Jenkins. Please take a seat until the doctor can see you. May I have your insurance card? Please put this thermometer [1]_____.

Patient:　(*coughing*) OK.

Nurse:　　Mr. Jenkins, you can go in now.

Doctor:　 Our nurse tells me your temperature is 102°F. That's a little high. [2]_____ are you experiencing?

Patient:　I've had a fever for two days, and my whole body feels sore. I'm really tired too, and I can't [3]_____.

Doctor: Hmm. Let me check ⁴_____. Yes, your throat is inflamed. Hold still, please. I want to listen to your chest. Take a deep breath.

Patient: OK. (*Patient starts coughing*)

Doctor: Did you ⁵_____ last fall?

Patient: No, I didn't.

Doctor: You have a mild case of the flu. Drink fluids so that you don't become dehydrated, and get some rest. Avoid exertion for 24 hours. Please get this prescription filled next door. It will ⁶_____ coughing so that you can get some rest.

III Reading Activity

次の英文を読んで、設問に答えなさい。

Health Insurance in the United States

Many people in the United States cannot afford to purchase basic health insurance. According to the US Census Bureau report of 2002, 38 million people were not covered by any form of health insurance. Even with insurance, medical procedures, operations, exams, and prescribed medicines are very expensive. Dental work is not included with basic medical insurance.

Typically, members of a group health insurance plan can expect to pay a hefty annual deductible, and then pick up 20% of the tab for every doctor's visit or procedure. Individual insurance on a non-group plan may easily cost $500 a month for someone aged 50 or older. Since most physicians will insist that patients undergo various expensive procedures and exams so that the doctor can provide as comprehensive a diagnosis and prognosis as technology will allow, a basic diagnosis of an illness is not cheap.

Is it any wonder that many older Americans are turning to alternative health care? Natural herbal remedies and teas, exercise, and a more nutritious diet are believed by many to promote and maintain physical well being, thereby reducing the number of times when it is necessary to go to a doctor. For those who must take medicines on a regular basis, the lure of cheaper priced drugs in Mexico and Canada continues to attract millions of Americans, who can purchase the same medication at a greatly reduced cost. According to a recent report from the American Association for Retired People (AARP), 73 million Americans traveled south of the border to buy their drugs last year.

■NOTES■

US Census Bureau　アメリカ商務省(Department of Commerce)の管轄下にある国勢調査局

group insurance plan　団体保険

pick up the tab for　費用を負担する

American Association for Retired People　アメリカ退職者協会。退職した人たちの生活のために活動する非営利団体（non-profit organization）

■Comprehension Questions■

1. Why don't many Americans have health care insurance?

2. Why do physicians want their patients to take many diagnostic tests?

3. What kind of health care is becoming more common in the US? Why?

4. What does AARP stand for?

5. Where did 73 million Americans go to purchase their medications last year?

IV Writing Activity
今まで学習した表現を参考にして、次の日本語を英語になおしなさい。

1. 他にどのような症状がありますか。

2. それを飲むと咳を抑えられます。

3. 来年は、インフルエンザのワクチンを受けられることをお勧めします。

V For Your Information
次にあげる病名または、語句を調べなさい。

1. leukemia
2. malignancy
3. sarcoma
4. bulimia
5. otitis media
6. diverticulitis
7. incontinence
8. plantar wart
9. renal (adjective)
10. lymphoma

NOTES

1) アメリカの医療保険制度は日本の医療保険制度と大きく違っています。例えば、日本の医療保険制度のもとでは、出産後、1週間ほど入院します。しかしながら、drive-through delivery という言葉があることからもわかるように、アメリカでは出産直前に入院し、出産の24時間後には退院するということが珍しくありません。ちなみに、分娩室は delivery room、妊婦さんに「踏ん張って」と言う場合には、push を用います。出産は大変なことから、labor という語が用いられます。

2) アメリカの新聞において「緑茶」の効用が大きく報じられたこともあり、以前にもまして緑茶への関心が高まっています。その記事では、1日1杯の緑茶を飲むことで、心臓発作や胃癌、腎臓癌の危険性が44％もさがると指摘されています。これは、緑茶に含まれるポリフェノールが酸化防止の働きをもつためです。

3) インフルエンザのワクチンは、日本では、注射により接種しますが、アメリカでは鼻孔からスプレーするものもあります。

Chapter 10

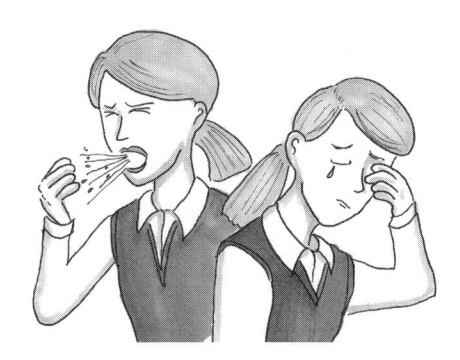

I Vocabulary Study

次にあげる英語表現の意味を表す日本語を選択肢から選んで、その記号を答えなさい。

1. intolerance ( )   a. 吸収する
2. infancy ( )   b.（喘息などで）ぜいぜい息をする
3. antihistamine ( )   c. 幼少期
4. drowsy ( )   d. 食品添加物
5. wheeze ( )   e. 不耐性
6. absorb ( )   f. 抗ヒスタミン剤
7. food additives ( )   g. 眠気を誘う・眠い

CD 21/22

II Listening Activity

会話文を聞いて、空欄に英語を書き入れなさい。ただし、最初の1回は、テキストの文を見ないで、聞いてください。

Doctor: Good morning, Mrs. Duncan. It looks like your allergies [1]_____ again.

Patient: (sneezing) Yes. I feel awful. I can't stop sneezing. My eyes [2]_____ and I feel very itchy, too.

Doctor: The pollen count is very high. You have hay fever, a seasonal allergy. Do you have any [3]_____?

Patient: Actually, I had some trouble last night. My husband heard me wheezing and said I should come see you.

Doctor: Let me listen to [4]_____. I will prescribe an antihistamine for you.

Patient: Thanks. Will the medicine ⁵_____?

Doctor: You will probably feel a little drowsy. ⁶_____ in the evening. Take care, Mrs. Duncan. You should be feeling better very soon.

III Reading Activity
次の英文を読んで、設問に答えなさい。

Food Allergies and Food Intolerance

Many people suffer from various food allergies. This is a reaction to a particular food or food group that can range from mild to extremely severe. A food allergy may show itself during infancy. The first symptom may be a skin rash or nausea. While many people are mildly allergic to nuts, shellfish, chocolate, peanuts (legumes), shrimp, wheat, or eggs, a small percentage of people develop extremely severe allergies to these foods. In serious cases, the allergy can cause a sudden drop in blood pressure and can cause a person's throat to constrict (to close up). This life-threatening condition requires immediate emergency treatment and hospitalization.

Food intolerance is not the same as a food allergy. Food intolerance may be caused by a lack of an enzyme that is needed to digest a particular food. Lactose intolerance, for example, is the inability of some people to absorb lactose, a compound found in milk.

Some food additives are known to cause allergic reactions. These compounds used to preserve food may trigger headaches or rashes in some people. In particularly severe cases, food additives may cause migraine headaches.

The only way to prevent an allergic reaction to a food that causes a negative reaction is to avoid that food. Since it is not always clear what ingredients are used in prepared foods, people who suffer from specific food allergies must be very careful when eating out or buying take-out meals.

■ Comprehension Questions ■

1. What are some common food allergies?

2. What is the first symptom of a mild food allergy?

3. What is food intolerance? Give an example.

4. What is one purpose of a food additive?

5. How can someone who is allergic to a food prevent a reaction?

IV Writing Activity
今まで学習した表現を参考にして、次の日本語を英語になおしなさい。

1. くしゃみやかゆみ、それになみだ目というのは、花粉に対する反応です。

2. 抗ヒスタミン剤を処方しましょう。

3. 恐らく少し眠くなるでしょうから、夜に処方するようにしてください。

V For Your Information

次にあげる病名または、語句を調べなさい。

1. bone marrow
2. nephritis
3. stye (hordeolum)
4. cirrhosis
5. Caesarean section
6. medical record
7. typhoid
8. pernicious anemia
9. Guillain-Barre Syndrome
10. staphylococcus

NOTES

1) アレルギー反応に苦しむ人にはハーブが効果的であると考えられています。甘草の根（licorice root）は、アレルギー反応による炎症に効果があることがわかっていますが、血圧上昇につながる場合も考えられるため、処方には注意が必要です。甘草（カンゾウ）の根に加えて、ゴボウ（burdock）、イチョウ（ginkgo）、タンポポ（dandelions）なども花粉症によるアレルギー反応に効果があると考えられています。

2) 外国人は納豆（natto）を、「拷問にかけられるように絶えられないにおいを放つ豆（odoriferous soybeans to torture）」などと表現し、納豆のにおいが嫌なようです。また、納豆は、molded beans とか steamed soybeans that are fermented とか紹介されていますが、実際にはそれがどのようなものか理解できない外国人が多くいます。しかしながら、鉄分、ビタミンB2、B12やたんぱく質を多く含むことから非常に栄養が高い食べもの（nutritious super-food）として紹介されるようになりました。また、コレステロールを多く含まない（lower cholesterol）食べ物で、結腸癌（colon cancer）、乳癌（breast cancer）、前立腺癌（prostate cancer）の予防や骨粗しょう症（osteoporosis）に効くものとして紹介されるようになっています。

Chapter 11

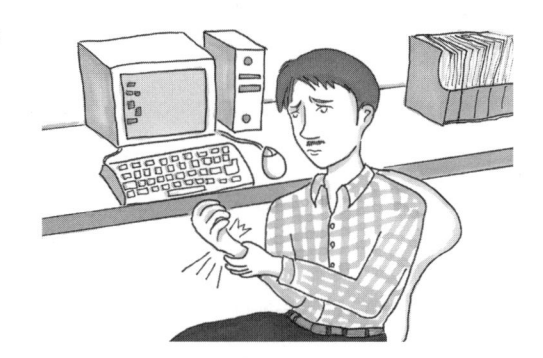

I Vocabulary Study

次にあげる英語表現の意味を表す日本語を選択肢から選んで、その記号を答えなさい。

1. Carpal Tunnel Syndrome ( )   a. しびれ
2. flex ( )   b. 手根管症候群
3. numbness ( )   c. （腕・膝などを）曲げる
4. persist ( )   d. （予想以上に）持続する
5. shooting pain ( )   e. （手足などに走る）ずきずきした痛み
6. nerve ( )   f. 神経
7. tingling ( )   g. （ひりひり・ちくちく）痛む

CD 23/24

II Listening Activity

会話文を聞いて、空欄に英語を書き入れなさい。ただし、最初の1回は、テキストの文を見ないで、聞いてください。

Doctor: What can I help you with today?

Patient: Well, Doctor, something is wrong [1]_____. When I flex it, it really hurts. The pain seems to shoot up my arm.

Doctor: Let me check. Hmmm. [2]_____?

Patient: Yes, that hurts.

Doctor: Do your fingers and hands [3]_____?

Patient: My right hand feels a little weaker than the left.

Doctor: [4]_____ do you spend using your computer?

Patient: Oh... about five hours.

Doctor: Have you been playing much tennis recently?

Patient: I play three times a week. Last Sunday I had to _____ because my wrist hurt so much, and I didn't have any strength.

Doctor: You have [6]_____, often referred to as CTS.

III Reading Activity
次の英文を読んで、設問に答えなさい。

Carpal Tunnel Syndrome

Repetitive motion may cause the tissue inside a nerve channel to become inflamed. The major nerve that carries signals from the brain to the hand travels through a rigid channel, or tunnel, formed by the wrist bones (the carpals). The swelling tissue presses on the nerve traveling through the wrist causing pain, numbness, or a tingling "pins and needles" sensation. This condition is known as CTS.

A similar condition may occur in the ankle and foot when the posterior tibial nerve is constricted. This is called tarsal tunnel syndrome. The symptoms are a burning sensation and numbness in the soles, toes or calves. If the condition persists, an operation is sometimes necessary. The compressed nerve is freed by creating more space in the tunnel.

The condition also occurs frequently among both sports players and artists who often use repetitive motions. Pregnant women are also susceptible to CTS. Doctors believe that hormonal changes in pregnant women may cause water retention, resulting in swollen wrists as fluids build up.

■Comprehension Questions■

1. What is CTS?

2. What are some of the symptoms of CTS?

3. What activities might cause CTS?

4. From this reading, we can infer that tarsal must be related to what body part?

5. How can surgery relieve the pain of CTS?

IV Writing Activity
今まで学習した表現を参考にして、次の日本語を英語になおしなさい。

1. 痛みは、腕全体に広がっていくようなひどい痛みを伴うものですか。

2. 手や指に力がはいらない状態ですか。

3. 私の診断では、CTSと呼ばれている手根管症症候群です。

V For Your Information
次にあげる病名を調べなさい。

1. cervical
2. hematuria
3. retch
4. corn
5. laceration
6. metastasis
7. enteric
8. food poisoning
9. gallstone (cholelithiasis)
10. renal failure

NOTES

1) 1980年代初期ごろまでは、CTSは、同じ作業を繰り返し行う仕事に従事する人々（ピアニスト、タイピスト、削岩機・チェインソーを用いる人等）だけに見られるものと考えられてきました。今日では、コンピューターの普及にともなって、いろんな職種の人に見られるようになっています。

2) アメリカでは、CTS予防としてコンピューターを使用する場合は、フォントが大きい文字を用いるように薦めています。フォントが小さい場合は、背を丸めてモニターを見るようになるため、首・肩・腕などの神経に必要以上の力がかかるためです。また、軽いタッチのキーボードを用い、強く打たないといけないものは避けるように薦められています。

3) 肩こりは、stiff shoulder/neckと表現します。日本語における肩は、shoulderとneckを含む語です。

Chapter 12

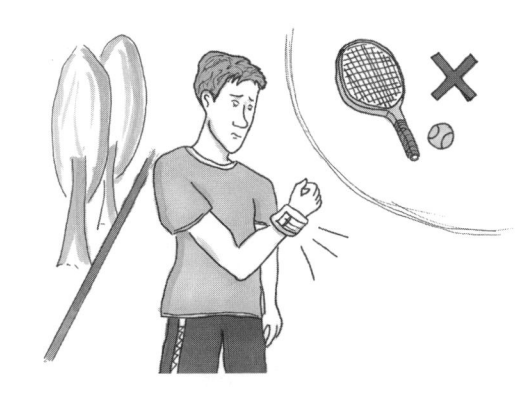

I Vocabulary Study

次にあげる英語表現の意味を表す日本語を選択肢から選んで、その記号を答えなさい。

1. sprain   (   )   a. 菌性の
2. fracture   (   )   b. 骨折
3. immobile   (   )   c. （手首・くるぶしなどの）捻挫
4. pad   (   )   d. 当て物
5. fungal   (   )   e. 強くする・強化する
6. nerve entrapment(   )   f. 神経にさわる症状
7. splint   (   )   g. 動けない・固定した
8. strengthen   (   )   h. 副木

II Listening Activity

会話文を聞いて、空欄に英語を書き入れなさい。ただし、最初の1回は、テキストの文を見ないで、聞いてください。

Patient: Doctor, what can I do about this Carpal Tunnel Syndrome? It's really painful.

Doctor: Don't worry. CTS is ¹_____ these days. People who spend a lot of time working on the computer are at risk. Also, ²_____ you use when playing sports can cause it.

Patient: Well..., I can stop playing tennis for awhile!

Doctor: I'm going to give you a special pad and splint to attach to your wrist. The splint will keep ³_____. Use it

Patient: when you use your computer.
Patient: Do I just put it on my wrist like this?
Doctor: Yes. Also, here's a handout with some diagrams of wrist exercises. I want you to do these ⁴▆▆▆ twice a day.
Patient: OK. Thanks. No more tennis for awhile, right?
Doctor: That's right. Stay away from tennis for now. ⁵▆▆▆ to come back in a couple of weeks.
Patient: Thanks, Doctor. See you in two weeks.

III Reading Activity

次の英文を読んで、設問に答えなさい。

Sports Related Injuries and Conditions

Fractures and sprains are common injuries related to sports activities. A sprain is a sudden twisting of a joint that can tear the ligaments. Anyone who has had a sprain knows how painful it is. A fracture is a break in a bone, in which the surrounding tissue is also injured. The skin surface above the break is sensitive to touch and often swollen or bruised. Fractures usually require surgery.

    It is now recognized that excessive racquetball, tennis, or any repetitive motion may cause Carpal Tunnel Syndrome (CTS). Using a special pad or splint, and refraining for awhile from the repetitive motion sport that caused the nerve entrapment can heal CTS.

    Other common sports related conditions are otitis externa, or "swimmer's ear," and "athlete's foot," or tinea pedis. Although both are minor ailments, they are unpleasant. Swimmer's ear, an infection of the external ear canal, is caused by prolonged submergence in water. It is usually treated with antibiotic eardrops. Athlete's foot is a contagious fungal condition, easily picked up in a gym or indoor pool locker room, where the fungus thrives. Many people suffer from this unpleasant fungal infection of the feet which causes great discomfort, blistering, and itching of the toes.

■NOTES■
otitis externa　外耳炎
tinea pedis　水虫

■Comprehension Questions■

1. What is the difference between a sprain and a fracture?

2. What is the physical cause of CTS?

3. Otitis externa is more commonly known as _____. What is it?

4. What causes "athlete's foot"?

5. What are the symptoms of "athlete's foot"?

Ⅳ Writing Activity
今まで学習した表現を参考にして、次の日本語を英語になおしなさい。

1. CTSは、最近よく見られる症状です。

2. 手首の関節を強化する運動を1日2回行ってください。

3. テニスは差し控えてください。

V For Your Information

次にあげる病名または、語句を調べなさい。

1. Buerger's Disease
2. heart failure
3. myocardial infarction
4. climacteric
5. malformation
6. flat foot
7. excessive acid secretion
8. mandible
9. olfaction
10. frozen shoulder

NOTES

1) canは、単なる推量を表すmayとは異なり、ある理論的、あるいは証拠に基づいた推量を表します。アメリカで販売されていたタバコのラベルは、"Smoking may cause cancer." から、"Smoking can cause cancer." へ変化し、因果関係がはっきりしてきた今日では "Smoking causes cancer." と記されています。

2) アメリカでCTSかどうかを自己診断（self-test）する方法として、"Phalen's Maneuver" が紹介されています。先ず、左右の手の甲を合わせて腕をまっすぐ前方に伸ばします。そして肘と手首ができるだけ直角になるように曲げながら、手を胸元に引き寄せます（写真参考）。このとき痛みを感じるのであればCTSの可能性が高いことになります。痛みを感じる場合は、60秒以上この動作を持続してはいけません。

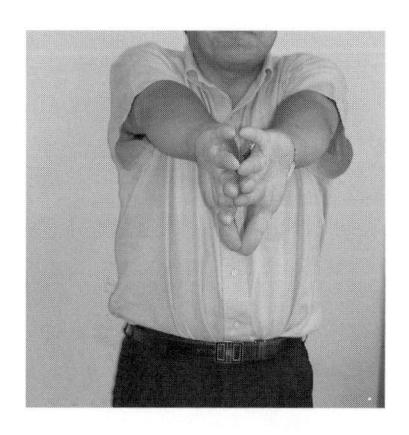

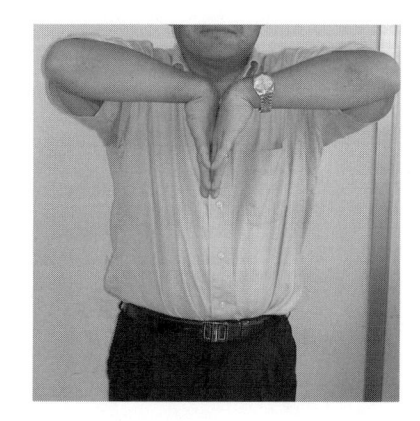

Chapter 13

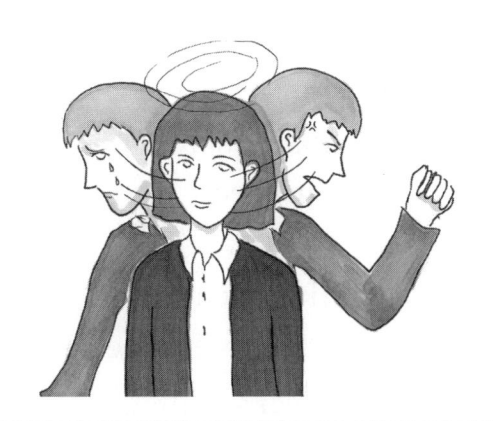

I Vocabulary Study

次にあげる英語表現の意味を表す日本語を選択肢から選んで、その記号を答えなさい。

1. estrogen   (   )
2. having a period   (   )
3. hot flash   (   )
4. ovaries   (   )
5. osteoporosis   (   )
6. ovulation   (   )
7. progesterone   (   )

a. 卵巣
b. 月経期を迎える
c. （更年期障害等による）皮膚の紅潮
d. エストロゲン（卵巣からでる女性ホルモン）
e. 骨粗鬆症
f. 排卵
g. プロゲステロン

CD 27/28

II Listening Activity

会話文を聞いて、空欄に英語を書き入れなさい。ただし、最初の1回は、テキストの文を見ないで、聞いてください。

Doctor: Good morning, Mrs. Jenkins. Time for your annual pelvic checkup, isn't it?

Patient: Yes, Doctor. I also need to talk to you about something.

Doctor: ¹_____?

Patient: Well..., my periods have been so irregular in the past eight months. Could I ²_____ menopause?

Doctor: That's very likely. Describe some of the other symptoms you are experiencing.

Patient: I'm a lot moodier, ³_____, and more irritable than usual. I often feel dizzy. I don't know why I feel so fatigued.

Doctor: ⁴_____ like classic menopause symptoms. Have you had any hot flashes?

Patient: Oh, yes. I'll feel hot and ⁵_____ in a sweat, and then I feel a chill. ⁶_____ and wake up perspiring.

Doctor: OK. After your pelvic exam, we'll run a little hormone test. I think that you have started menopause.

III Reading Activity

次の英文を読んで、設問に答えなさい。

The Change of Life

Menopause, often referred to as the "change of life," is a significant change for a woman as it marks the ending of her cyclic menstruation periods. Childbearing years end when the ovaries no longer produce eggs. Menopause is not simply a physical condition. As the amount of estrogen and other sex related chemicals change, a woman may experience both physical and emotional disturbances. The ovaries release less and less estrogen and progesterone and in time, the ovulation stops. Though the average age of menopause is fifty, the "change of life" may occur at any age between the mid-thirties and the early fifties. Menopause may begin gradually with irregular menses, or menses may stop abruptly from one month to the next. How women respond and react to this change is unpredictable and varies from individual to individual. Some women experience no emotional sensitivity and few physical symptoms, other than the cessation of their periods. Other women suffer from a variety of symptoms that include hot flashes, irritability, nervousness, and pain during intercourse.

Until recently, HRT, or hormone replacement therapy, had been very popular in both Europe and the United States. The purpose of HRT is to replace lost hormones with natural or synthetic estrogen and progesterone. It was widely believed that this treatment not only alleviated the discomfort many women felt, but that it also protected them from serious health problems in the future. Lack of estrogen and hormonal imbalance in postmenopausal women puts them at a much greater risk for osteoporosis and cardiovascular diseases, both major health concerns for older women.

New medical research indicates that HRT does not do all that women were promised. In fact, some studies link long term use of HRT to greater incidences of Alzheimer's, heart disease, and various cancers. For this reason, many women are discontinuing HRT and are looking for natural ways to relieve symptoms and keep their hormones in balance.

■NOTES■
HRT or hormone replacement therapy　ホルモン置換療法
postmenopausal　閉経後の

■Comprehension Questions■

1. Why do you think menopause is sometimes called "the change of life"?

2. What is the physical cause of menopause?

3. Do all women who experience menopause have the same symptoms?

4. What is the purpose for HRT?

5. Why is HRT a controversial treatment for menopause?

●Chapter 13

IV Writing Activity

今まで学習した表現を参考にして、次の日本語を英語になおしなさい。

1. どうやら更年期障害の症状みたいですね。

2. ふだんよりも物忘れをしたり、いらいらしたりしますか。

3. 骨盤の検査をした後に、ホルモンテストをしましょう。

V For Your Information

次にあげる病名または、語句を調べなさい。

1. cataract
2. infertility
3. pharyngitis
4. deafness
5. metabolism
6. SIDS
7. goiter
8. smallpox
9. miscarriage
10. hysterectomy

NOTES

1) 日常会話では、メンスを迎えた女性は、I became a woman. と表現する場合もあります。

2) 英語圏では、アジアの人々は大豆類や緑茶を多く摂取し、中南米の人々はヤマノイモ (yam) を摂取しているので更年期障害がひどくないと信じられています。まだ詳しいことは明らかではありませんが、更年期障害の度合いには食事が深く関係し、中でもイソフラボノイドが関与しているのではないかと考えられています。

3) 最近、アメリカでは、日本の老人ホームにあたる施設で、ペットと入居することが許されるようになっています。これは、老人がペットと時間を過ごすことで、孤独感 (loneliness) や気分の沈滞 (depression) から免れたり、また、散歩したりすることで血圧の上昇を抑えたり、ストレスを解放するなどの効果が報告されているからです。

4) アメリカ人の平均寿命 (life expectancy) は、76.9歳で、女性は79.5歳、男性は、74.1歳です。最近の報告では、60歳を迎えた人のうち400万人ほどの人が痴呆 (dementia) の症状が見られ、なかでもアルツハイマー病 (Alzheimer's disease) の割合が多く、記憶障害 (memory loss)、言語障害 (language loss) などで苦しんでいます。レーガン前アメリカ大統領もアルツハイマー病にかかり、そのことを公表しました。

Review Test 2

🎧 CD 29

Part 1 LISTENING EXAM　英文を聞き、次の質問に答えなさい。

■■■ Comprehension Questions ■■■

1. This conversation is taking place _____.
    A. in a doctor's office
    B. in a hospital
    C. on the telephone
    D. on email

2. The woman is talking to the doctor about _____.
    A. her son's health
    B. her daughter's health
    C. her own health
    D. her mother's health

3. Lucy feels _____.
    A. energetic
    B. lethargic
    C. sleepy
    D. active

4. Lucy's mother thinks Lucy looks _____.
    A. pale and thin
    B. strong and healthy
    C. overweight
    D. depressed

5. What does the doctor NOT mention?
    A. anorexia
    B. anemia
    C. diabetes
    D. depression

6. The doctor wants to give Lucy a _____ test.
    A. urine
    B. blood
    C. psychological
    D. cardiovascular

7. We can infer that low iron levels may indicate _____.
    A. anemia
    B. appetite loss
    C. anorexia
    D. changes in weight

8. The mother is going to take Lucy to the doctor _____.
    A. this morning
    B. this afternoon
    C. tomorrow morning
    D. tomorrow afternoon

| Part 2 READING EXAM | 次の英文を読んで、設問に答えなさい。 |

Flu Shots

Influenza is a serious medical condition that affects the respiratory system. Some of the symptoms are fatigue, muscle soreness, fever, a sore throat, and congestion. Although most people recover in a few days, the immune system of some older patients is so weakened that the flu can lead to pneumonia. More than 110,000 people are hospitalized with influenza each year in the US, and an average of 36,000 people die from complications caused by the flu. Because the virus that causes influenza changes each year, the US Center for Disease Control and Prevention (CDC) recommends new shots be taken each year by everyone over the age of fifty. Millions of people across the US go to community centers to get the flu vaccine in autumn before the beginning of flu season.

Recent research indicates that people who get annual flu shots may be receiving other benefits. In a study of 286,000 people aged over 65 who had the flu shot, hospitalization for heart disease and strokes dropped by nineteen percent and sixteen percent, respectively. For those who had taken the flu shot for two consecutive years, statistics show an even greater drop in hospitalizations for these serious illnesses. Health officials remind the public that the flu vaccine does not prevent SARS, the serious respiratory disease that killed 800 people in 2003.

■NOTES■
US Center for Disease Control and Prevention (CDC)　アメリカ疾病予防局

■■■ Comprehension Questions ■■■

1. Influenza is an illness that primarily affects the _____ system.
    A. circulatory
    B. cardiovascular
    C. intestinal
    D. respiratory

2. Some elderly patients with the flu may develop pneumonia if they have _____.
    A. a high fever
    B. great fatigue
    C. a weak immune system
    D. sore muscles

3. According to the passage above, we can infer that most Americans get their flu vaccine in _____.
    A. January and February
    B. May and June
    C. October and November
    D. March and April

4. It is advisable to get a new flu shot each year because _____.
    A. the flu virus changes each year
    B. the benefits wear off in a year

　　　　　C. the vaccine improves each year
　　　　　D. the vaccine prevents SARS
5. Most people who have the flu are hospitalized.
　　　　　A. True　　　　　B. False
6. Approximately one third of patients hospitalized with the flu in the US die.
　　　　　A. True　　　　　B. False
7. New research indicates that flu vaccine seems to help prevent heart disease.
　　　　　A. True　　　　　B. False
8. Two hundred and eighty six thousand people over the age of fifty participated in the recent study referred to above.
　　　　　A. True　　　　　B. False
9. Taking flu shots for two years in a row did not improve chances for not being hospitalized for a stroke.
　　　　　A. True　　　　　B. False
10. Another benefit of the flu vaccine is that it reduces the possibility of contracting SARS.
　　　　　A. True　　　　　B. False

Part 3 VOCABULARY EXAM 1～10の英文に合う最も適切な語句を選択肢から選んで、答えなさい。

1. The young woman felt tired and _____. She had little interest in anything and was unable to get her work done.
　　　　　A. olfaction　　　B. lethargic
　　　　　C. exertion　　　D. routine
2. The symptoms of _____ are often described as severe pains in the wrist.
　　　　　A. CTS　　　　　B. SIDS
　　　　　C. AIDS　　　　D. RMD
3. With a weakened _____ system, the body is less resistance to infections.
　　　　　A. drowsy　　　　B. anemic
　　　　　C. olfactory　　　D. immune

4. To repair a fractured bone or to heal CTS, a doctor may have the patient wear _____.
   A. an ice pack   B. a Band-Aid
   C. a splint   D. an iris

5. In the spring and fall, trees and plants release _____ that may activate allergies for many people.
   A. pollution   B. pollens
   C. smells   D. insects

6. During _____, a woman's menstrual periods are irregular and she may experience hot flashes and other uncomfortable symptoms.
   A. menses   B. menopause
   C. ovulation   D. miscarriage

7. One way to _____ your body is to exercise regularly.
   A. stronger   B. practice
   C. strengthen   D. weaken

8. During a _____ annual checkup, a doctor checks a patient's blood pressure and weight.
   A. routine   B. extension
   C. cyclic   D. birth

9. High amounts of _____ in the body can result from a diet high in fats and may cause a stroke or a heart attack in time.
   A. calcium   B. cholesterol
   C. pollen   D. blood

10. _____ surgery is very common for elderly people whose vision has become blurred and cloudy with age.
    A. Carcinoma   B. Iris
    C. Cataract   D. Visual

11. Many people in the United States cannot afford to buy health _____.
    A. investigation B. insurance
    C. prescription D. subscription

12. A patient needs to describe his/her symptoms to the doctor for an accurate _____.
    A. diagnosis   B. hormone
    C. diagonal   D. pediatrician

症状集

Respiratory symptoms （呼吸器官の症状）
1) I have a fever.
2) I have a stuffy nose.
3) I have a runny nose.
4) My tonsils are swollen.
5) I have a wheezing cough.
6) I cough a lot.
7) I gargle, but the pain in my throat doesn't go away.
8) I have a sore throat.
9) I cough up phlegm.
10) I feel tired / worn out / drained.
11) I'm not sleeping well.
12) I have insomnia.

Cardiovascular symptoms （心臓血管の症状）
1) I have a squeezing pain here.
2) I feel pressure in my chest.
3) When I go up stairs, my heart begins to pound / palpitate.
4) I sweat a lot.
5) Sometimes I am out of breath.

Headache symptoms （頭痛の症状）
1) I have a migraine headache.
2) My head hurts on this side.
3) My head is pounding.
4) I've got a tension headache.
5) I feel a headache coming on.

Gastrointestinal symptoms（胃腸の症状）
1) I have a stomachache.
2) I doubled over when I felt a sharp pain in my stomach.
3) I have a chronic/acute pain in my stomach.
4) I have diarrhea.
5) I have loose stools.
6) My stomach seems to be bloated. Also, I feel bloated.
7) I feel nauseous.
8) I have heartburn.
9) I am suffering from a bad case of constipation.
10) I can't eat. Everything makes me sick.

Skin symptoms（皮膚の症状）
1) I have a rash all over my body/my stomach/my arms.
2) My skin is itchy.
3) I have dry skin.
4) My skin is too oily.
5) I have acne.
6) I have too many pimples.
7) I break out in hives when I eat (strawberries / tomatoes / shellfish).

Eye symptoms（目の症状）
1) My eyes are itchy.
2) My eyes are watery.
3) I am suffering from dry eyes.
4) My right eye is red.
5) My eyes are gummed shut with eye mucus.
6) My eyes feel tired/sore.
7) I feel like something is in my eye, but I can't see it.

Ear symptoms（耳の症状）
1) My hearing is going.
2) My ears are ringing.
3) My ears feel congested.
4) My ears itch.
5) I have an earache.
6) I think I need to get the wax removed from my ears.
7) I've got water in my ear. I went swimming without a cap / Swimmer's ear. (I've got "Swimmer's ear")

Musculoskeletal symptoms（筋骨格の症状）
1) I sprained my ankle.
2) My face / arm / shoulder / thigh is bruised.
3) This morning I had cramps. (I've got cramps now)
4) My arm aches when I stretch it.
5) I twisted my ankle / wrist.
6) Something is wrong with my hand / arm / neck / shoulder / etc.
7) My arm / neck / shoulder / hand / knee feels very sore and tender.

表現集

Before Examination（診察前）
1) What seems to be your problem?
   (*or* What's brought you here today?)
2) What symptoms do you have?
3) How long have you had this problem?
4) Do you have any other symptoms?
5) Did anything special bring it on?
6) Please describe the pain.
7) Do you have pain anywhere else?
   (*or* Do you have any other pain?)
8) What's your normal temperature?
9) Are you taking any medicine regularly?
10) Do you take any medicine?
    Did you take any medicine (before...)?
11) Are you allergic to any medication?
12) Have you ever had a rash on your body due to any medication? What about penicillin?
13) Do you have a sore throat?
14) Does your throat feel rough?
15) Have you been wheezing?
16) Do you have a dry cough?
17) Have you coughed up any phlegm?
    ("Phlegm" is more commonly used than "sputum.")
18) Can you describe the phlegm? Is it very thick?
19) What color is the phlegm?
20) Have you had swollen tonsils before?
21) Do you feel pain when you swallow?
    (*or* Is there any pain when you swallow?)
22) Have you ever been told your thyroid is swollen?
23) Is your face often puffy?
24) Do you have a persistent/oppressive/throbbing pain in the chest?
25) Do you have heartburn?

26) Do you have a feeling of discomfort in your stomach?
27) Do you feel nauseous?
28) Do you have a good/poor appetite?
29) Do you feel abdominal pain when you're nauseous?
30) Do you have soft stools?
31) Do you feel a sharp pain in the lower abdomen?
32) Is this the first time you have had a convulsion?
33) Are you getting enough sleep and nutrition?

In the Examination Room（診察室にて）

34) I'd like to examine you. Please undress from the waist up and put on this robe.
35) Take a deep breath. In. Out.
36) Open your mouth. Put your tongue out, and say "Ah."
37) Hold your breath.
38) Lie face down. (Lie on your stomach.) Turn to your left/right side.
39) Let me take your pulse and blood pressure. 140 over 95. It is a little high for your age.
40) Let me take your temperature. Keep the thermometer under your arm.
41) Let me check for an abnormal change in your heart rate.
42) We need a sample of your blood and urine for lab tests.
    We need a stool sample.
43) We'll need to take an electrocardiogram.
44) You'll need a chest X-ray.
45) You'll need to have some tests to see how your liver and kidney are functioning.
    (*or* You'll need to take some liver and kidney function tests.)
46) We'll give you a local anesthetic.
47) We'll give you some antibiotics.
    We'll prescribe some pain killers.
48) We'll give you some mouthwash.
49) I'll give you an antacid.
    I'll give you indigestion medicine.

50) When was the last time you had a mammogram (cholesterol test / chest X-ray / etc)?
51) Please complete this family health history form.
52) How much do you smoke per day? How much do you drink in a week?
53) Have you recently gained/lost any weight?

人 体 図

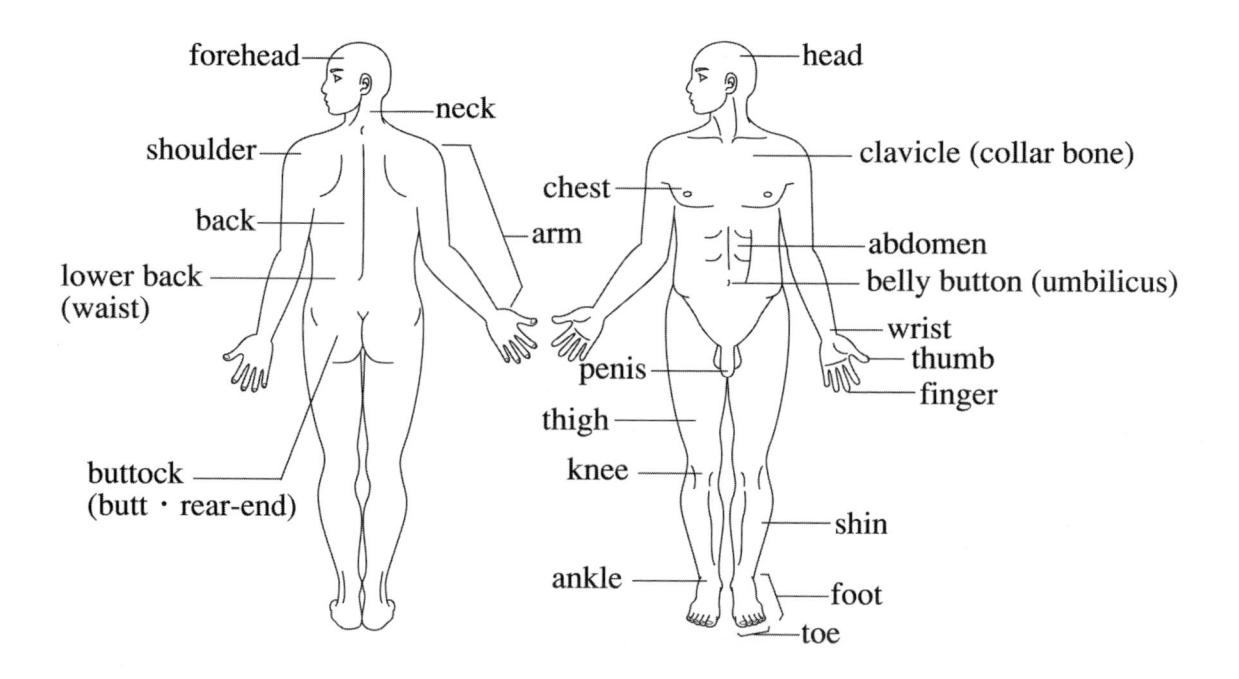

- forehead
- neck
- shoulder
- back
- arm
- lower back (waist)
- buttock (butt・rear-end)
- head
- clavicle (collar bone)
- chest
- abdomen
- belly button (umbilicus)
- wrist
- thumb
- finger
- penis
- thigh
- knee
- shin
- ankle
- foot
- toe

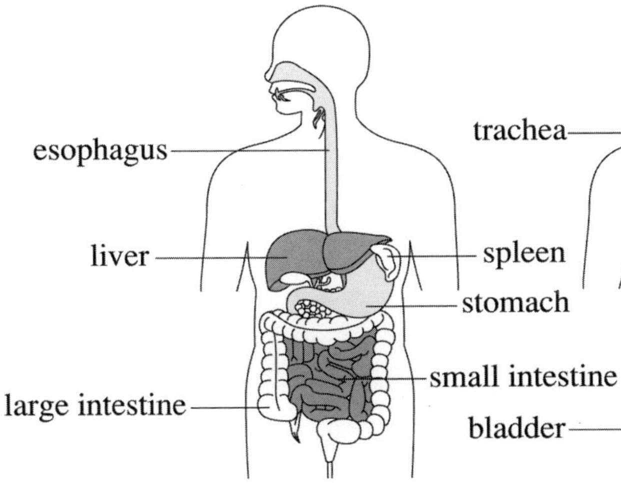
esophagus
liver
spleen
stomach
small intestine
large intestine

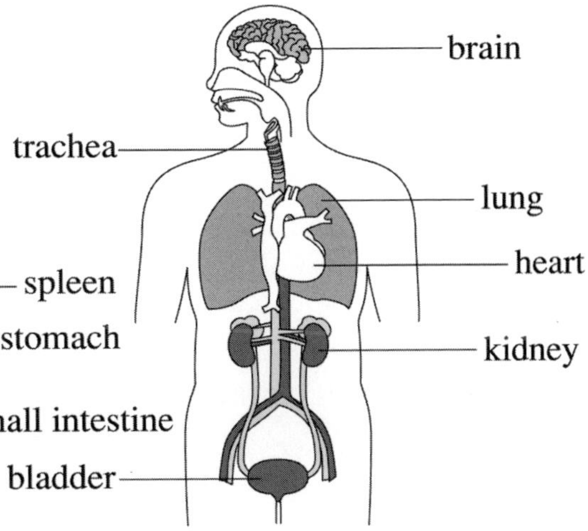
brain
trachea
lung
heart
kidney
bladder

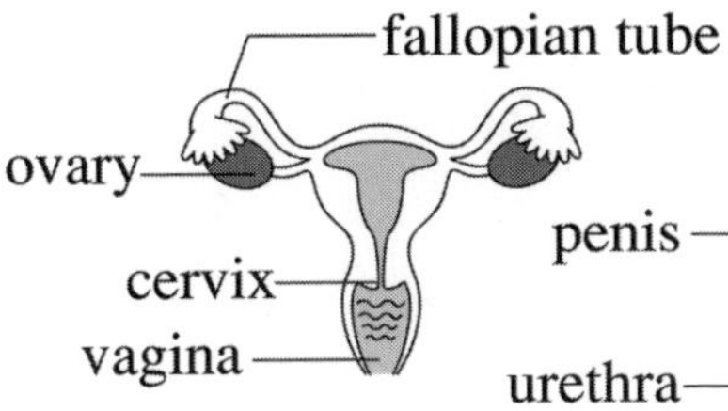
fallopian tube
ovary
cervix
vagina

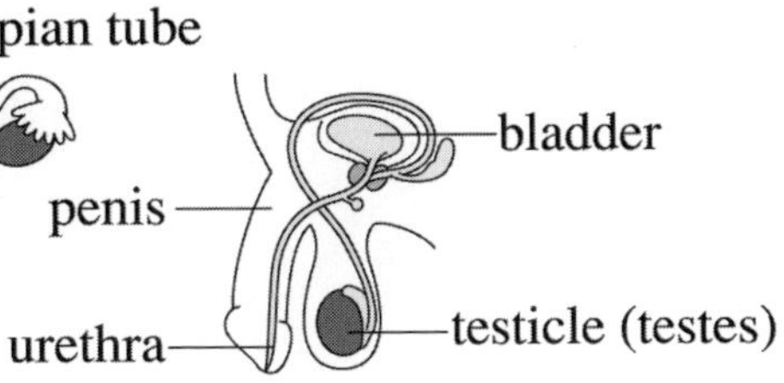
bladder
penis
urethra
testicle (testes)

本書にはカセットテープ（別売）があります

English for Medicine
―医療・看護のためのやさしい総合英語―

2005年1月20日　初版発行
2020年9月30日　重版発行

著　者　　　　西　原　俊　明
　　　　　　　西　原　真　弓
　　　　　　　Assunta Martin
発行者　　　　福　岡　正　人
発行所　　株式会社　金　星　堂

（〒101-0051）東京都千代田区神田神保町3-21
TEL: (03) 3263-3828　　FAX: (03) 3263-0716　　振替: 00140-9-2636
URL: http://www.kinsei-do.co.jp　　e-mail: text@kinsei-do.co.jp

編集担当／佐藤求太
印刷所／倉敷印刷　製本所／松島製本　1-7-3805
本書の無断複製・複写は著作権法上での例外を除き禁じられています。本書を代行業者等の第三者に依頼してスキャンやデジタル化することは、たとえ個人や家庭内での利用であっても認められておりません。
落丁・乱丁本はお取りかえいたします
ISBN978-4-7647-3805-8 C1082